Case Histories From a Successful

Naturopathic Clinic

Healing Chronic Illnesses Naturally

by

Dr. Earendil M. Spindelilus D.N.M., M.H., C.R., PSc.D

DISCLAIMER

This book is intended to provide information on the subject of chronic diseases and possible alternative care. This information presented is not intended as a substitute for medical training or advice, but every effort has been made to ensure accuracy.

The book is sold on the understanding that the publisher and author are not liable for any misconception or misuse of the information provided and shall have neither liability nor responsibility to any person or entity with respect to any loss, damage or injury caused or alleged to be caused directly or indirectly by the said information.

Table of Contents

CHAPTER FOUR CHRONIC

CHAPTER FIVE INCURABLES

DEDICATION

To my wife and best friend Peggy, who has stood beside me and put up with all of my time spent getting one degree or certification after another.

To Waya and Sinde, our furry children who love us unconditionally.

I would also like to express my gratitude for all of the patients who have taught me so much about how to be a doctor.

Not all doctors are healers and not all healers are doctors.

Introduction

The purpose of this book is to offer hope for an alternative treatment for chronic disease. The information contained describes in a small detail some of the work and case histories I have personally witnessed in my 20+ years of practice as an alternative healthcare provider. You will find a wide variety of cases ranging from simple cuts and wounds to serious auto-immune disorders such as Multiple Sclerosis and type 1 diabetes along with successful treatments for cancer.

You will notice as a common theme throughout each of these cases an overriding need for cleansing and dietary and lifestyle changes. This displays a single important point for ridding our bodies of disorder, cleansing it and making the appropriate changes so we do not end up back in the old condition. It is interesting to note that a survey was done by the AMA of all physicians who treat cancer. It was a one questions survey.

Each physician who had cancer patients in remission was to ask their patients if they had changed their lifestyles or diet having "survived" cancer. Even the AMA was stunned at the results. Over 90% percent came back and stated that they had not changed their lives in any manner. Hence, the reason cancer has a return rate of about five years and usually with a vengeance. This is actually not unexpected when you realize that only 6% percent of all U.S. physicians have had even a single semester credit of nutritional education out of eight years of higher education. That leaves us with 94% of all U.S. physicians with no education in nutrition, even though congress mandated that they receive said education. Today only half of all medical universities require this course.

It is in part because of this lack of knowledge on the doctor's behalf that illness continues to spread in the World's wealthiest nations. According to Clinic Compare out of Britain, they analyzed 179 countries based on information from the World Health Organization. America is the only non-European country to make the top 10 on the list, having the ninth highest rate of obesity in the world — 35% of the adult population is classified as dangerously overweight. It is considered the sickest nation in the developed World. As well as from other studies the results surprised even the researchers. To their alarm, they said, they found a "strikingly consistent and pervasive" pattern of poorer health at all stages of life, from infancy to childhood to adolescence to young adulthood to middle and old age. Compared to people in other developed nations, Americans die far more often from injuries and homicides. We suffer more deaths from alcohol and other drugs, and endure some of the worst rates of heart disease, lung disease, obesity, and diabetes.

Among the most striking of the findings are that, among the countries studied, the U.S. has:

- The highest rate of death by violence, by a stunning margin

- The highest rate of death by car accident, also dramatically so

- The highest chance that a child will die before age 5

- The second-highest rate of death by coronary heart disease

- The second-highest rate of death by lung disease

- The highest teen pregnancy rate

- The highest rate of women dying due to complications of pregnancy and childbirth

According to Pure Wellness out of the U.K., the United States has one of the worst diets in the World. As stated on their website:

"…where every portion of food or drink can be 'super-sized'. This is the world of plenty! But where did it all go wrong for this nation? According to the documentary, it all started back in 1971 where President Nixon was hopeful for a re-election. Many Americans at the time were very unhappy about the high cost of food. So to get the price down, Nixon encouraged farmers to mass produce crops......and one in particular—**corn!** This process created a new product called **high fructose corn syrup (HFCS)**—A cheap sugar sweetener that can be found in thousands of food products today. However, it didn't just stay in America. This processed product spread like wild fire to other countries with similar dieting problems such as... ".

Stress levels are also on the rise. A recent report shows America to be among the most stressed out nations on Earth. People are becoming more and more disconnected from the natural world and spending their lives in an environment devoid of tress, grass and open, quiet spaces.

So, what can be done about it? We need to take back control of our own lives and start caring for ourselves. As some wise folks have said in the past "Start eating like an adult". Start making healthy choices for yourself and that can start with a vegan diet. Organizations such as the World Health Organization, The U.N., Kaiser Permanente, the American College Of Lifestyle Medicine, The Physicians Committee for Responsible Medicine, Academy of Nutrition and Dietetics, The Mayo Clinic and many, many more recommend a plant-based diet.

We can also start looking for more natural alternatives for treating our selves and out families. While it is slowly increasing in the U.S., countries such as in Europe have been using herbal medications for thousands of years. To this day, you can go to a pharmacy in England and half of it will be pharmaceuticals and the other half stocked in natural medications. Physicians in Germany will prescribe St. John's Wort 90% of time over Prozac while the opposite is true in the States. Germany was so interested in proving the efficacy of herbal medications that their equivalent to the U.S. FDA funded a massive research project called the German Commission E. This study proved the efficacy of 380 different herbal substances.

Within these pages you will find holistic medicine's tried and true protocols used successfully for each and every type of condition. Whether I have a patient come in with a cold or cancer I basically treat them the same. Our clinic has gown throughout the years to being the most successful holistic clinic in Northern California because we follow Dr. Christopher's recommendations. Over the years I have seen thousands of patients and cannot take the time to list all of the wonderful people I have met. I will try and cover some of the more memorable here in this book. The names have been changed to protect their medical privacy.

CHAPTER 1

Accidents

1.1 Peggy Knives

You will notice several case histories detailing a particular patient by the name of Peggy. I must say that she is both my wife and my Herbal Poster Child. She has probably given me more practice than any patient in my 16 year history. This particular case history details a couple of very serious wounds.

Case History #1 Knife wound:

One afternoon my wife was at the house while I was with patients at the clinic. She had finished washing the dishes and they had been drying in the dish drain, yes, some folks still do that.

When the time came to put the silverware away she reached and grabbed several at the same time. Within the group was a knife pointing downward. While she was moving to the drawer the knife slipped out and embedded itself into her exposed foot.

She looked down and saw the knife sticking straight up with a little blood seeping from the point of impact. She knew as soon as she removed the knife the blood would flow. Fortunately, she kept the cayenne tincture we had made nearby. She removed the knife and the blood began to spurt from the wound.

She immediately placed about a dropper full of the tincture on her tongue and noticed within 30 seconds that the bleeding came to a stop. While the cayenne may be very hot it causes no tissue damage and it can be a very successful treatment for bleeding.

Case History #2 Vegetable slicer:

About a week prior to the previous event Peggy was slicing up a zucchini for my meal. Again, I was not at home but her having graduated from the Family Herbalist course prepared her for emergencies such as this one.

While slicing the vegetable she grew impatient. With only a slice or two remaining to be done she removed the blade guard to speed up the process. The very next slice removed a significant portion of her thumb at the tip. This produced a heart beat spurting of blood from the wound.

She immediately ran and retrieved the cayenne from our medicine shelves. She orally took about a dropper full and also poured some of the cayenne tincture on the counter and rubbed the wound in it. Needless to say, the pain was significant, but again, no tissue damage.

As she watched, the blood flow rapidly diminished and within about 60 seconds it had slowed to a gentle ooze.

1.2 Peggy - Burns

Again we return to my favorite patient, my wife Peggy. This event occurred due to an extremely overheated wax women use for their bikini area.

As usual, I was not at home when this occurred but due to her education with the School of Natural Healing she knew what to do.

She was microwaving wax and left it in too long. She had also been using the same plastic container for years and it had degraded. When she pulled the wax out of the oven the bottom collapsed and the molten wax poured onto her leg and foot.

The resulting effect was a second degree burn, just shy of third degree. She knew to immediately get the B, F and C salve out of the refrigerator and tried to apply it to the burn but unfortunately the wax had seared to the flesh and could not be removed.

She called me and I rushed back to the house. I found her on the floor in pain. I helped her into the living room where I then applied a very generous amount of the salve straight onto the top and surrounding area of the wax. Within minutes the salve began to seep under the wax and the pain diminished.

Within about 40 minutes enough of the salve had worked it's way under the wax and we were able to simply lift it off of her foot. Underneath was a very serious deep burn. We applied more salve and over the next two weeks she would reapply it and bandage.

In the end, the burn completely healed with no lasting scarring. Needless to say, that was the end of waxing.

1.3 Bob - Gangrene

This was most likely the worst case of gangrene with extensive tissue necrosis I have ever had to treat. I had treated this patient in the past for various simple issues and had not seen him in about eight months. He called me on a Sunday requesting I make a house call as soon as possible. He stated he had damaged his foot back in November of the previous year and it was now early January.

I arrived at his house to find a foot in the early stages of gangrene. The flesh had begun to turn red, phasing towards brown. He had an elevated temperature and a rapid heart beat. The foot had become greatly swollen with an extensive flow of pus and lymph from the small wound on the bottom pad. The smell in the house was almost unbearable.

He stated the original wound was from a simple tack stepped on in the back yard that Fall. Something told me to check his blood sugar. I had never treated him for diabetes but I went ahead and checked. He had a blood glucose level of 300. Here we had a very serious situation of uncontrolled diabetes. He was in great danger of losing his foot as well as going into septic shock.

He stated he would not go to the hospital so we began treatment on the spot. I cleaned the wound and began applying herbal antiseptics. The formula used we call Herbadyne, the herbal sister to Betadine. It contains Myrrh, Goldenseal and Cayenne. It does sting just like Iodine. After this we dressed the initial wound in B, F and C salve.

For the systemic infection, we put him on Garlic at five capsules every hour. We also included the formula **Infection** from Dr. Christopher at the same dosage. He was also given Echinacea/Goldenseal at 4 capsules 4 times a day.

He was also instructed to eat as much raw garlic each day as he could stand, usually in the form of Dr. Christopher's Flu Stew. The Blood Stream formula was also administered each day at 4 droppers 5 times a day to cleanse the infection from his blood.

To aid in rebuilding the massive tissue loss, both skin and muscle, he was instructed to take B, F and C at 5 capsules 5 times a day.

To combat the gangrene, he was to soak his foot in an Epsom bath with a decoction of Marshmallow and Lobelia two to three times a day, soaking for a half hour or more. B, F and C fomentations were also used at night. During the day, the same salve was kept on the bottom of the foot.

After about a month the wound on the bottom of the foot began to seal but the infection was far from over. With nowhere for the infection to go the body found a way. Skin eruptions began to occur on the top of the foot. The patient and his wife called them little volcanoes. They could watch the eruption swell over the course of a day and then finally they would burst and the infection would literally flow out. It was the **Blood Steam** formula which aided in finding an avenue for the infection to leave the body.

Around the second month we began to apply a plantain poultice to the top of the foot where the eruptions where occurring. He was to continue with the previous treatment except the new poultice was to be kept on all night. This finally turned the tide and the infection began to diminish.

All told, it took about three months for the greater part of the healing to occur. The patient and his wife had stated to me, due to past experience with other family members, that if we had not followed the type of treatment protocol, a hospital would have removed several toes, if not the entire foot. Below are a serious of pictures demonstrating the healing.

His recovery has been a blessing. Because of the extensive use of the B, F and C he noticed that his old back injury was healed and can now even lift weights again. His diabetes also shows signs of healing as he is now completely off his diabetic medication.

Be warned, they are graphic.

The first week of treatment
Initial wound

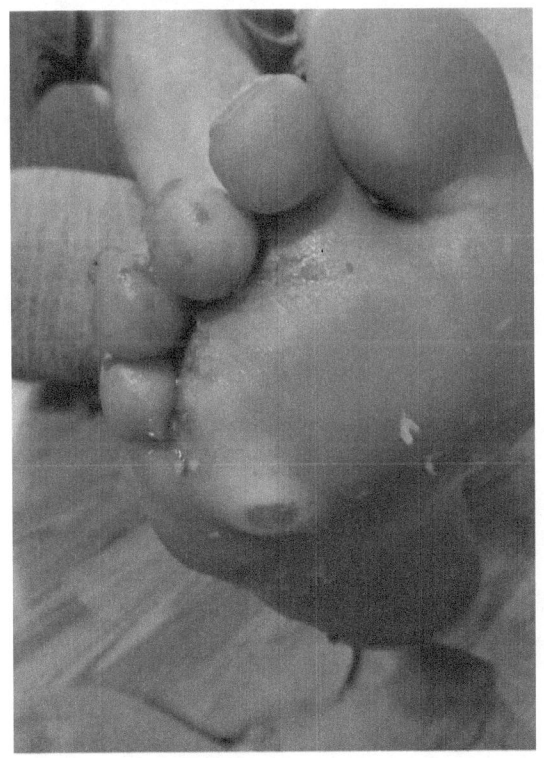

The First Month

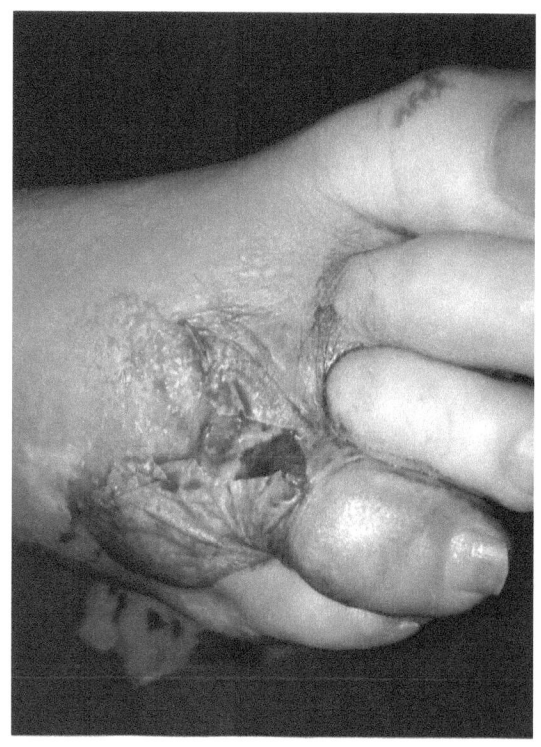

A closer look

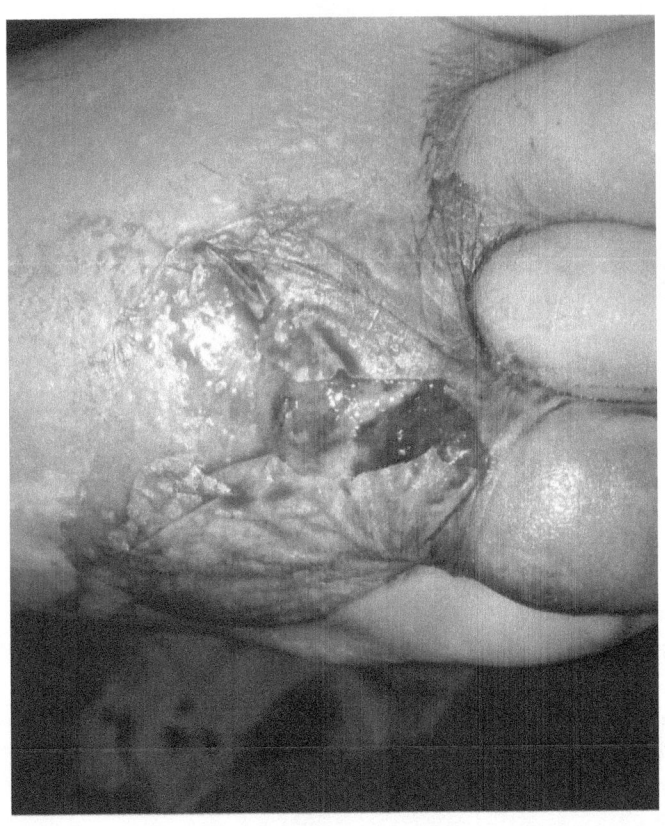

Two months into treatment

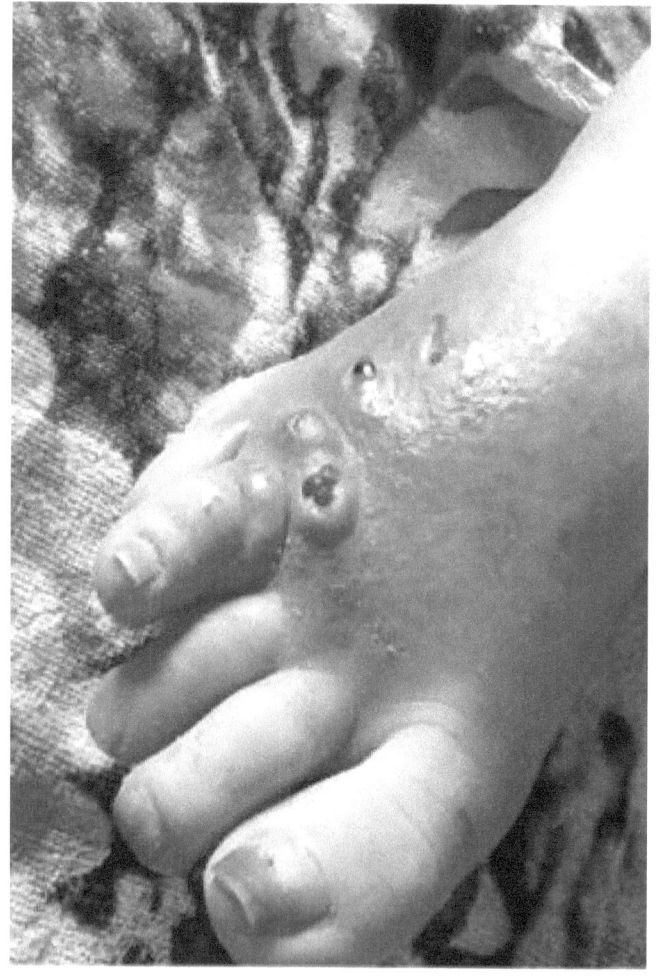

First Week of May

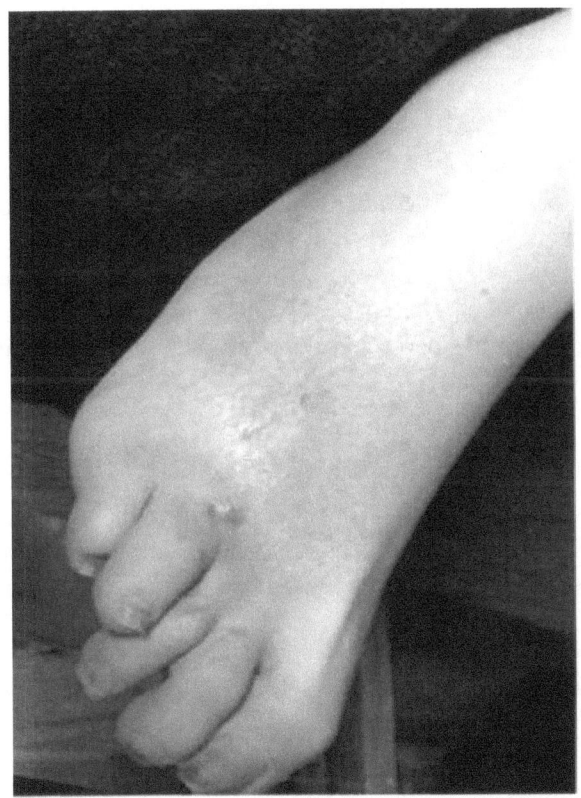

CHAPTER 2

Children

2.1 Jill – Pregnancy

This has to stand out as one of the most wonderful and moving cases I have had in reference to pregnancy. Jill is a current patient with the clinic and originally came to us to treat her children for such minor issues as colds and bronchitis. Then one day she announced she was pregnant and wanted us to assist in the pregnancy to insure a healthy baby and delivery. She currently uses a midwife and plans for a home water delivery.

One morning she called the clinic during her 11th week and stated she was spotting. We asked her to immediately come in. Upon arrival we had a very distraught mommy to be and we did a basic exam over the abdomen and listened for the baby. At this point we did not see anything wrong so we ran an ultrasound to check on the child. The joy in her face when we showed her a bouncy baby with a strong heartbeat made the rest of my week a happy one.

We still were not sure what was causing the bleeding so we dispensed to her Dr. Christopher's Anti-Miscarriage formula consisting of False Unicorn and Lobelia. Within twenty four hours she reported that the bleeding had stopped. What she reported next was nothing short of a miracle.

Within the first day or two of using the formula she felt something passing through her cervix. A small bean sized, gel encased sack was expelled which she promptly took to her midwife. The midwife informed her it was an eight week old fetus that had passed and that Jill had been carrying it alongside the healthy fetus.

The anti-miscarriage formula had caused her to expel the fetus which had passed several weeks earlier, while saving the healthy fetus. Currently, she is having a very healthy pregnancy and is still taking the anti-miscarriage formula.

17 Mar 2015   Tree Of Life Holistic Wellness Center

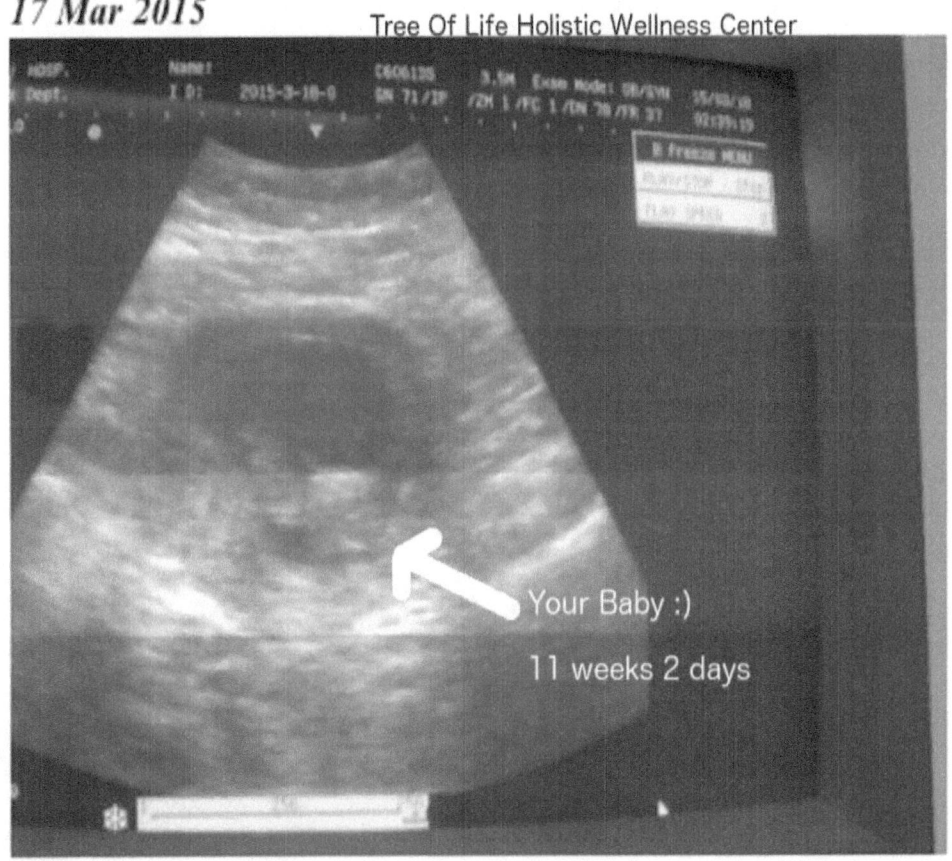

Your Baby :)

11 weeks 2 days

2.2   Jane – Pregnancy

Jane is one of those cases that you will remember for the rest of your life as it contains the gift of new life. She came to us shortly after I had started my career as a Master Herbalist. She had been told she could never have a child as she could not safely carry to term.

We told her there is no such thing as an incurable disease and that nothing was written in stone. She started the incurables program with a mucous-less, vegan diet and began using the Formulas **Lower Bowel**, and **Liver and Gallbladder** while drinking plenty of Red Raspberry tea.

We also put her on the formulas Female Reproductive and Hormonal Changese with wheatgerm oil. Prior to starting the herbal therapy she also did the three day cleanse using carrot juice. We find carrot juice one of the best liver cleansers in nature.

After about eight months on this program we recommended that if she chose to she could try again to become pregnant. She did in fact become pregnant quick quickly and nine months later gave birth to a beautiful little boy.

He is now about 14 years old and a gift to us all.

2.3 Mark – Impotent

This patient was actually a nephew in law and came to us with an issue of impotency. I knew him as a small child and he was one of those constantly picked on by his other cousins. When full grown he was quite tall and had decided he was no longer going to be abused. It was at that time he started taking steroids, synthetic testosterone. In the end he became a very large and muscular man. The ladies loved him.

Eventually he met the love of his life and they married. After about a year of marriage his wife asked him to stop taking the steroids as she knew they were very dangerous and put him at risk for such diseases as prostate and testicular cancer among a wide variety of other issues. He did as she asked.

This resulted in a complete lack of sex drive nor the ability to perform sexually. As we were taught at the School of Natural Healing, if you give the body something it should be making on it's own, it will stop making it. This resulted in the atrophying of the testicles and their shrinking.

We had him do a three day cleanse with carrot juice and stated the basic program using **Lower Bowel, Liver and Gallbladder, Blood Stream** and the glandular formula continuing Mullein and Lobelia.

Due to the severity of his case he was also told to use the Mullein and Lobelia as a fomentation directly on his testicles each night for six nights a week for many months. This was quite embarrassing for him as it required the use of a cloth diaper held in place while he watched TV each night.

I asked them to not try and have a child for at least one year. The wife also followed the basic program and ate better during this time.

In time he did heal and they were able to conceive and have a little baby girl.

2.4 "Cub" - Severe bronchitis

"Cub" was a six month old little boy who came into the clinic with sever bronchitis. This past Winter we saw so much of this we named it the "crud". It would always start as a simple cold and then progress into the chest.

We took his vitals and he did have a small fever and quite a bit of discharge from the sinuses. Since he was still breast-feeding we asked the mother to take garlic at a dosage of 4 capsules five times a day. For "Cub" we had her administer to him a dropper of Dr. Christopher's formula **Lung and Bronchial** along with the **Super Immune Garlic** extract. Children seem to do quite well with the flavor of both of these formulas.

We also instructed the mother how to do the onion poultice with olive oil on his little chest, to be done each day. The formula Sen Sei was also applied each day to aid in his breathing.

Within about two days he was showing remarkable recovery and in a week the issues were over.

UPDATE:

A few months later he came into the clinic with a serious issue of constipation. He had not had a bowel movement in four days. We asked the mother to give "Cub" the children's version of the liquid **Lower Bowel** and asked her to use it at a dosage of half a dropper twice a day. I told her to expect results within twenty-four hours.

She reported that after an hour of the first administering, done at the clinic, he had a very successful bowel movement and was much more regular from that point on.

2.5 John - Appendicitis

"John" was a nine year old boy with acute appendicitis. His parents had originally taken him to the hospital with sever pain in the lower right quadrant of his abdomen. He was diagnosed with acute appendicitis and was advised to have immediate surgery. The family had a serious financial issue and also did not believe in removing his appendix.

They called me late at night and requested our help as an emergency situation. They had pulled him out of the hospital and met me at the clinic.

We opened the clinic for them and made sure they understood the seriousness of the situation and asked if they were sure this is the path they wanted to take. They again requested our assistance so we began to treat him.

W immediately began to administer the formulas **Lower Bowel** and **Liver and Gallbladder**. We also asked the parents to administer catnip and fennel enemas which brought immediate relief from the pain.

For the rest of the night we had them use castor oil packs over the appendix area using the twelve minutes hot and four minutes cold routine. This also aided in relieving any pain the child was experiencing.

By the end of the night the pain was completely gone and the issue had passed. The parents later had him checked out and no sign of the appendicitis could be found. Yet another appendix saved from the surgeons knife.

2.6   Multiple Autism cases

We have had multiple cases of autism brought into our clinic over the past several years. I have little doubt that vaccines are the leading contributing factors behind these issues. No child that came into our clinic who has never received vaccines have we ever seen this issue present.

At our clinic we are able to run a urinalysis test for neurotransmitters. We can test for six different transmitters and this gives us a very clear understanding of what is happening within the brain. The test results for all autistic children are almost identical. They almost invariably show a significant imbalance in the chemicals of the brain, leading to OCD, attention disorders and a lack of social skills.

Our standard protocol utilizes a mucous-less diet, cleansing routines using the formulas **Lower Bowel** and **Liver and Gallbladder** . With this we add the following formulas **MindTrac** (or **Kid-e-Trac**), **Relax-Eze** and **St. John's Wort.**

Invariably, within a two month period of the children following the program we receive reports of the children's moods stabilizing, their attention spans increasing and the ability to sleep better at night. One particular mother reported to us that she felt she had her son back. We will go into this issue in greater detail when we discuss Nathan who had both psoriasis and autism.

2.7 Lisa – Morbid obesity and Pregnancy

This was a very rewarding case which stands as proof that even those patients with a high risk pregnancy can have a healthy and vibrant child. Our patient was a 24 year old female who was morbidly obese at 300+ pounds. She originally came to us with Polycsytic Ovarian Syndrome and was unable to conceive. We put her on the standard holistic program for female reproductive issues utilizing such herbal medications as Blessed Thistle, Red Raspberry tea, Black and Blue Cohosh, as well as colon and liver cleansing routines and a vegan diet.

She had issues with loosing weight due to a high stress life and turning to food for comfort. But, over time she did lose some of the weight and eventually did conceive. At this point no other doctor would work with her as she was considered such a high risk case. Morbid obesity during pregnancy can commonly lead to gestational diabetes causing the baby to become too large, placenta previa, high blood pressure and miscarriage, to name just a few.

We continued to treat her and to support the pregnancy. She stayed on at least a quart a day of Red Raspberry tea. I know that a simple search of the web gives grave warnings of drinking Red Raspberry tea during pregnancy but it is not true. All of our pregnant patients are put on this tea and have seen amazing results with a healthy pregnancy and babies.

We also put her on an anti-miscarriage formula utilizing False Unicorn and Lobelia. In an earlier case in this book I discuss the wonderful benefits of this formula and have never seen it fail in preventing miscarriage.

We monitored her throughout her pregnancy with blood work and ultrasounds each month. She remained on the vegan diet and after nine months delivered a beautiful baby girl and throughout her pregnancy did not have a single complication, as would have been predicted by most obstetricians.

2.8 Johnny – Almost fatal anemia – age 21 months

Sometimes a case will come to us that moves our hearts and stays with us long after the patient has been treated. This is a case of a very little boy who came very close to death with little advanced notice to his parents.

I received a call on our emergency line a Friday when the clinic was closed. It was from a very distraught mother calling from UC Davis fighting not to lose custody of her child to the hospital. Earlier that morning the child walking tough the house when he suddenly collapsed and was unable to move one side of his body. The parents immediately rushed him to the local hospital where they examined him and ran a blood test. The blood test revealed a hemoglobin level of a 4, a very dangerous level when a normal level for him would be more in the 12 range. The hospital evaced him down to US Davis oncology.

After receiving him, the hospital determined he needed an immediate blood transfusion. His parents are Jehovah's Witnesses and transfusion are against their faith so they declined. At this point the hospital notified them that if they refused they would remove the child from their custody and perform what procedures they felt necessary. The mother, whose mother and father were both patients of ours, called and asked for us to intervene to stop their child from being taken away from them.

I spoke with the hospital and told them I would take over the care of the child with the agreement that we would send weekly blood test results to them. Amazingly, they agreed. I spoke again with the mother and gave him some basic advice for the weekend and to bring him into the clinic on Monday. Since I was not sure what was the cause of his condition I asked for them to at least get him started on organic black strap molasses, a food extremely high in calcium and iron. We also had his blood test results sent to me immediately so I could review the case.

One of the most common mistakes many doctors make with anemia is the diagnosis that the patient is low on iron. This is actually usually not the case but simply one of a lack of assimilating the iron already present in the blood. What the blood test results revealed was a surprise to me. The child was actually in iron overload and the lab showed he was already experiencing kidney and liver damage. High iron in the blood can cause both liver and kidney damage. Originally, the hospitals thought it was a viral infection, which can cause these types of symptoms in little ones. A more detailed intake done at our clinic revealed that the mother had given him too may iron supplements, resulting in iron overload. If the hospital had given him the transfusion it most likely would have killed him, since he already had too much iron in his system resulting in kidney and liver damage.

We kept him on the black strap molasses and also started him on a dietary routine high in the minerals that better enable to the body to assimilate iron. We also also put him him on a natural, herbal iron formula. Again, this was not necessarily high in iron but in the minerals and vitamins required to assimilate what was already in his little body.

Each week we checked his hemoglobin levels and faxed them to UC Davis. Each week they continued to rise and within four weeks he was at normal levels. Almost immediately, his skin color improved as well as his energy level and he was quickly back to a very energetic 21 month old little boy.

CHAPTER 3

Lung Issues

3.1   William – COPD

William was an 89 year old patient with severe COPD and was dependent on an oxygen bottle to survive the night. He also required a rescue inhaler and various other asthma type medications.

He stated he was ready to get away from these medications as he knew they were very damaging to his liver. As always, we never have a patient get off of their medicaments as this could be very dangerous. We let their previous primary lower their dosage as they notice they no longer need them as much. Eventually they are usually able to get completely off of them.

He started the mucous-less diet after a very successful three day cleanse with carrot juice. He followed the cleansing program using **Lower Bowel, Liver and Gallbladder** with **Kidney** and **Blood Stream** added later. We also added the Lung and Bronchial formula along with a tincture made from Mullein and Lobelia to act as a bronchial dilator and anti-spasmodic.

We also used the formula **Complete Tissue and Bone** to aid in healing the lung tissue. After about two months he was off the oxygen bottle and by month three all of his medications were discontinued.

To this day he has not required any of our formulas or the previous medications. An interesting note, it took him about five months to get the oxygen company to come and pick up the bottles as the company did not want to lose the insurance payments.

3.2   Paul – Tuberculosis

Paul is an immigrant patient from Mexico who came into the United States as a nine year old child. At that time a TB test showed he was a carrier and was not active with the disease. This had a multitude of ramifications for him in such areas as getting employment and citizenship. He brought in a blood test which proved he was infected.

He came to the clinic to see if we could help him remove this condition. As Dr. Christopher stated, "There are no incurable diseases, just incurable patients". At the clinic we live by this statement.

We put him on the mucous-less diet along with the standard formulas of **Lower Bowel, Liver and Gallbladder** and later the **Blood Stream** formula. We also directly treated his lungs using the **Lung and Bronchial** and **Complete Tissue and Bone formulas**. He also did the three day cleanse using carrot juice. We put him on a strong regimen of garlic to combat the latent bacteria.

After being on the cleansing diet and the formulas for three months we had him tested again and the results showed no signs of the tuberculosis bacteria. I told him to hold on to that lab as proof for the future.

3.3   Steve – Chronic Pneumonia/Bronchitis

Here is a case with a patient who had been suffering from a long term chronic case of bronchitis with multiple instances of pneumonia each year. This had been going on for about ten years. He had to keep a rescue inhaler with him at all times and was on strong bronchial pharmaceuticals. He was also was a chronic smoker and stated he was not able to stop.

As in other cases, we placed him on the mucous-less diet, of which he only partially followed. I stated the most important dietary change had to be a complete lack of any kind of dairy. This he was able to do.

We followed the standard recommended protocol from Dr. Christopher and had him start on the formulas **Lower Bowel, Liver and Gallbladder** , **Lung and Bronchial** and the **Complete Tissue and Bone** capsules. Later in the program we added the **Blood Stream** formula.

Over time he noticed that a significant amount of mucous began to expectorate from his lungs. The original color was very dark, almost black. As the program progressed the color changed to a green, then a lighter yellow to eventually clear. His breathing continued to improve and he was able to stop taking his respiratory medications along with the rescue inhaler. He was still smoking but had cut it down to half. In time he was able to quite smoking altogether.

When he started the program he could not hold down a job. After about six months his health had improved enough to where he was able to go back to his construction job. He works there to this day.

CHAPTER 4

Chronic

4.1 Ruth – Lyme Disease

One of the joys we get at the clinic is the opportunity to be one of the only Lyme-literate clinics in Northern California. It is a sad state to find how little is known about this disease and how poorly the CDC encourages information. It is terribly under reported due to the CDC requirements being absurdly high for what can be classified as Lyme disease. Fortunately we have Dr. Christopher's knowledge and that of Dr. Burascano, the worlds leading authority on Lyme Disease. He is also very open to alternative medicine as an option for treatment. He has treated over 11,000 patients worldwide.

Ruth is a common example of a patient with Lyme Disease. Rarely does the patient receive treatment shortly after being bitten by the deer tick as this creature is quite small and most patients will not even realize they have been bitten. In only 20% of the cases does the classic "target" rash show up. In her case she was not diagnosed until about nine years after he initial infection. This results in what we classify as chronic or late term Lyme Disease with secondary infections.

This usually results in chronic joint and muscle pain, fatigue, a suppressed immune system along with a variety of other symptoms. She had been constantly misdiagnosed and was usually labeled with Chronic Fatigue Syndrome, a blanket diagnosis meaning they have no idea what is happening to the patient.

In her case we finally received a blood test back called the Western Blot Test. It showed the bacteria markers for the Lyme Disease organism. We began treatment immediately. One of the most important things to do for chronic Lyme Disease is to deal with the long term damage which is usually with the nerves. We also have to be careful treating the disorder too aggressively as a large die-off of the bacteria can actually harm the patient.

We started with the three day cleanse using carrot juice and afterwards she adopted the mucous-less diet. The cleansing formulas **Lower Bowel** and **Liver and Gallbladder** along with the **Kidney** formula were also utilized.

To aid in the nerve and joint damage we also added the formulas **MindTrac, Relax-Eze, St. John's Wort, Complete Tissue and Bone** and the **Joint** formula. To aid in the compromised immune system we added the **Adrenal** Formula with **Immucalm.**

Within the first month on the program she noticed an increased energy and a lessening of the joint and muscle pain. Her physician in her area has asked for us to consult with him so he can better treat his other patients with this issue.

While this program usually takes about a year to complete she continues to improve to this day.

For those interested, we have a book published with Amazon titled _A Holistic Approach to Healing Lyme Disease._

4.2 Peggy – 92 prescription pills a week

Again we return to my wife Peggy. When we first got married I can say she loved me, just did not trust me with her health. She had been raised in the deep south where they tend to put physicians on a very high pedestal. This lasted for the first ten years of our marriage.

When we married she was on 92 prescription pills a week along with hip injects for a variety of different issues. She had extreme allergies to pollen and trees. She also had a very significant hormonal imbalance which left her in the fetal position every 28 days on the floor due to the pain of her periods. Her last condition was hypothyroidism, something they are told cannot be cured. She never did find relief from the pain or discomfort of any of her conditions while following conventional medicine.

After years of going to her physician she was told they give up and will schedule her for a full hysterectomy. The physician told her she was 36 years old and no longer needed her female organs. My wife had been with me long enough to know this was not a viable option. There are over 200,000 hysterectomies done in the United States each year and I do not believe any are necessary.

My wife had enough and asked me for help. I was overjoyed as I did not like seeing her in pain every 28 days. She was already a vegetarian so we cleaned her diet up a bit more and we started the program using **Lower Bowel, Liver and Gallbladder** and the **Blood Stream** as the cleansing components of the program.

For the allergies she started taking **Sinus-Plus** along with **Immucalm** and within a week her allergies were much improved. To this day she has never had the severe allergies from those days. Whenever a light attack occurs she simply takes a little **Immucalm** and **Sinus-Plus** again for a few days.

The hormonal imbalance required the use of the formulas **Female Reproductive, Hormonal Changese** along with Wheatgerm oil. She also started drinking about a quart of Red Raspberry tea a day.

The first 28 days rolled by and up came her first period on the program. While the pain was still quite severe she noted that it was somewhat less in intensity. All in all, it took about three months before she was able to happily declare she had her first normal period in life, in more than 20 years.

At this point now she was down from 92 prescription pills a week to just seven, for the thyroid. She was no longer having any hip injections. I asked her if she was ready to get rid of the hypothyroidism. The answer was a resounding yes.

For this issue it is important to feed and care for the Thyroid. We do this through the use of the formulas **Herbal Thyroid**, **Thyroid Maintenance** and **Kelp**. Mullein and Lobelia is also taken internally as a great glandular aid. During the later stages of the program we put a fomentation of the Mullein and Lobelia over the thyroid on her throat every evening before bed for six nights. It took another three months before she was off the last of the pills. It was getting close to the end of the year by this point so she decided to have a full blood panel done up by her old physician after the first of the year to see how she was doing.

When the results came back she was very pleased. It showed no sign of the allergies, hormonal imbalances or the hypothyroidism. Her physician looked at her and stated, in first person, "I guess I cured you". My wife walked out of there and never looked back.

A side note: 18 years later my wife entered menopause. Because she had already gotten her hormones in balance, menopause was not what most women in this country experience. There were no hot flashes, night sweats, changes in libido or vaginal dryness. Menopause is a gift meant to take a women from one phase of life to a more freer one. Unfortunately, most women in this country experience just the opposite.

4.3   Christine – High Blood Pressure

High blood pressure is epidemic in this country with prescription medication for it one of the highest recommended. We had a patient by the name of Christine who was on two of these types of drugs and was beginning to show liver issues. Even while on the medication her blood pressure remained constantly high.

We put her on the standard program with dietary changes, the three day cleanse and the cleansing formulas **Lower Bowel**, **Liver and Gallbladder** and **Blood Stream**. To aid the blood pressure issue directly we recommended the formulas **Hawthorne Berry Syrup** and **Blood Circulation**.

Within the first month her blood pressure began to drop to the normal range while still on her pharmaceuticals. By month two her blood pressure was beginning to drop still further and her other primary had to drop her dosage of the drugs, By month three her physician had to completely take her off of them as her blood pressure was dropping too low. Off the drugs her blood pressure was now within the normal range and we were able to take her off of ours and to this day she is on none of the previous drugs.

4.4   Susan – High Cholesterol/Triglycerides

Susan had one of the highest triglyceride levels I had ever seen. She was in the danger zone being around 2000 when the average patient should be no higher than 150. She loved her sweets and carbs and seafood. Her cholesterol was also very elevated.

As always, we recommended the dietary changes utilizing the three day cleanse with the mucous-less diet. The usual cleansing formulas were also incorporated. The **Blood Stream** formula was also very significant here as it helped clean her blood out as an aid to clear out some of the cholesterol. We added garlic and flax and kelp as well to drop these levels further.

We ran the usual labs to monitor her levels and for a while they did drop some but very slowly. One of things that can confuse a patient is when they get on a vegan diet and find that their cholesterol continues to rise. This can be from two basic issues. One is that the liver is most likely damaged and need some assist. Also, during one's lifetime, when the liver cannot detoxify enough of the poisons traveling through the body, it will basically "take a bullet" for you and store them.

When you go on a good cleansing diet the liver suddenly finds itself in a large supply of the needed nutrients to do the job and it will attempt to convert this backlog. This can come out as bile and quite a bit of damaged cholesterol or LDL. I always tell the patients that if they can be patient the levels will eventually drop.

To further aid this issue we added milk thistle to heal the liver from a lifetime of bad choices. Within about three months the liver had healed enough to drop her triglycerides levels to 600 and by the fifth month she came back with a clean bill of health. She was no longer in danger of liver or heart disease.

4.5   Jack – Near Sighted

It is always a pleasure to see a patient relieved of a crutch that they have been hanging on to for most of their life. Glasses are no exception to this rule.

Jack had been wearing glasses for many years and was ready to let them go. We had already been treating his daughter for a serious hormonal imbalance due to endometriosis at the age of 27 and then a hysterectomy so he was familiar with the program.

While he did not follow the program very well he still ended up with wonderful results. He barely made any dietary changes though he did try and stay away from dairy. He used the **Lower Bowel** and the **Liver and Gallbladder** formulas and added the formula **Herbal Eyebright** to his regimen. He used it twice a day externally and also used it internally.

Two months passed after using the formulas consistently he decided to go back to the DMV to take an eye test. He passed the test and the DMV removed the restriction from his license.

4.6   Virgil – Shingles and Heart Blockage

Here I get to return to a family member for a case history. This time it was for my father in law Virgil. When my wife and I married I was the foreigner (not from Alabama) who had come to take their daughter away from them. Needless to say, I was not well loved in that family.

About ten years into our marriage my wife and I opened our first clinic. Sometime after this Virgil called us and asked for help. Without us knowing it, he had been suffering from a very serious case of Shingles. This had been going on for about six weeks. His physician had to admit to him that he did not know what to do for him and asked if he knew of any old family remedies. It was at this time Virgil called us.

We immediately drove out to their house and found a man in such pain and misery. He was covered with the lesions from the top of his head and down his back and legs. We treated the shingles both topically and orally. Topically, we treated him with our formula called **Herbadyne** using Myrrh, Goldenseal and Cayenne. Internally, we treated him with high doses of Echinacea and Goldenseal root. Goldenseal is a wonderful antiviral. The dosage was five capsules five times a day.

By the next morning he called us and reported the pain was already diminishing and within a week the shingle's lesions were gone. I went from being the black sheep of the family to them going around church bragging about their son in law the doctor.

Two years later he called us again over another issue. His cardiologist found a 90% heart block and recommended open heart surgery. Virgil asked for a three month reprieve to try something different. The physician consented.

We knew he would not change his diet so we recommended a simply routine of distilled water and apple cider vinegar. This utilized mixing a glass of distilled water with a tablespoon or more of apple cider vinegar.

This was to be drank four times a day, six days a week. He was to follow this for the full three months.

After three months he went back to the physician and they canceled the surgery as the heart blockage went from 90% to 0%. He also experienced an interesting side effect from this program.

Before he stated the apple cider vinegar cleanse he had been unable to perform sexually for about 15 years. He happily reported that all systems were functioning once the vinegar had cleansed out all of the arteries.

4.7   Bestsy – Heavy Metal Toxicity

One of the most prevalent conditions in America today as well as in other industrialized nations is heavy metal toxicity. It is found in the food, the air, the soil, cigarette smoking and in the cloths we wear. Pharmaceuticals are filled with them such as mercury, aluminum, cadmium, lead and arsenic.

Some time back a 47 year old female patient came into our clinic complaining of a number of autoimmune type reactions as well as a serious candida and mold infection. During her intake we found that she was a potter and sculptor who made extensive use of glazing. Heavy metals can be found in the clay itself as well as the chemicals used for glazing. Her home also had a very serious mold problem. Her blood work showed infections and a hair analysis showed extensive heavy metals as can be seen by the following lab result:

TOXIC METALS		RESULT μg/g	REFERENCE INTERVAL	PERCENTILE 68th 95th
Aluminum	(Al)	8.1	< 7.0	
Antimony	(Sb)	0.12	< 0.050	
Arsenic	(As)	0.048	< 0.060	
Barium	(Ba)	4.0	< 2.0	
Beryllium	(Be)	< 0.01	< 0.020	
Bismuth	(Bi)	0.096	< 2.0	
Cadmium	(Cd)	0.12	< 0.050	
Lead	(Pb)	5.6	< 0.60	
Mercury	(Hg)	0.15	< 0.80	
Platinum	(Pt)	< 0.003	< 0.005	
Thallium	(Tl)	< 0.001	< 0.002	
Thorium	(Th)	0.002	< 0.002	
Uranium	(U)	0.014	< 0.060	
Nickel	(Ni)	0.29	< 0.30	
Silver	(Ag)	5.5	< 0.15	
Tin	(Sn)	1.1	< 0.30	
Titanium	(Ti)	0.57	< 0.70	
Total Toxic Representation				

She was very high in Antimony, Barium, Lead, Nickel and Silver. These metals are notorious for wiping out the intestinal flora and bringing bout a severe candida overgrowth, thereby compromising the immune system. This left her open to so many other co-infections such as mold and other bacterial types. Her original presenting complaints included candida and hormonal imbalances.

We stated her off with our standard candida cleanse, mentioned earlier in this document. This utilized a vegan diet due to it's low inflammatory nature and one low in natural sugar. She had to avoid all sugars and alcohol, even fruits for at least 18 days as well as use holistic medications for killing the candida, such as Black walnut and Pau'd Arco. We keep the bowels moving to help eliminate the dead yeast.

By the end of the 18 days she noticed a marked improvement in her thinking and level of energy. She proceeded to have the home cleaned out from the mold while we treated her for the mold in lungs, again, using the above mold and yeast formulas, but at a much lower dosage and for several months. She remained on the vegan diet as it is well established that the fiber and anti-oxidants and other chemicals in the plants help chelate the heavy metals from her body.

At this time we also prescribed a natural heavy metal formula called Dr. Christopher's Bugle Heavy Metal Formula. It utilizes Bugleweed, a known herb with a very strong history of success for removing heavy metals from the body. She remained on this program for at least six months. As each month passed on the program she felt her health improving which we conformed with blood work demonstrating the infections were disappearing. We finally ran another heavy metal hair test six months later. The surprising results are shown below:

TOXIC METALS		RESULT mg/g	REFERENCE INTERVAL	PERCENTILE 68th 95th
Aluminum	(Al)	3.6	< 7.0	
Antimony	(Sb)	0.035	< 0.050	
Arsenic	(As)	0.048	< 0.060	
Barium	(Ba)	1.5	< 2.0	
Beryllium	(Be)	< 0.01	< 0.020	
Bismuth	(Bi)	0.013	< 2.0	
Cadmium	(Cd)	0.046	< 0.050	
Lead	(Pb)	1.2	< 0.60	
Mercury	(Hg)	0.08	< 0.80	
Platinum	(Pt)	< 0.003	< 0.005	
Thallium	(Tl)	< 0.001	< 0.002	
Thorium	(Th)	0.001	< 0.002	
Uranium	(U)	0.020	< 0.060	
Nickel	(Ni)	0.12	< 0.30	
Silver	(Ag)	1.4	< 0.15	
Tin	(Sn)	0.14	< 0.30	
Titanium	(Ti)	0.34	< 0.70	
Total Toxic Representation				

As you can see from the above lab, the heavy metals showed a marked improvement which was mirrored in her improved energy levels, thinking and memory abilities and a total lack of bronchial and sinus issues.

She remains vegan to this day and is a shining example of a healthy and happy individual. We are all very proud of her.

CHAPTER 5

INCURABLES

5.1   Lilly – Utecarea

According to Wikipedia:

Urticaria (from the Latin *urtica* , "nettle" from *urere*, "to burn"), commonly referred to as **hives**, is a kind of skin rash notable for pale red, raised, itchy bumps. Hives may cause a burning or stinging sensation. They are frequently caused by allergic reactions; however, there are many nonallergic causes. Most cases of hives lasting less than six weeks (acute urticaria) are the result of an allergic trigger. Chronic urticaria (hives lasting longer than six weeks) is rarely due to an allergy.

The majority of chronic hives cases have an unknown (idiopathic) cause. In perhaps as many as 30–40% of patients with chronic idiopathic urticaria, it is caused by an autoimmune reaction.

In all of my career I have only had one patient with this condition. She was a 60 year old women with severe hives from the top of her head to the bottom of her feet. When she first came to the clinic all she could do was squirm in her chair while she related her story. It broke my heart to see her suffering so much. All the conventional medical establishment could do was to give her Prednisone.

Since it is an autoimmune condition we recommended the Incurables program from Dr. Christopher. She immediately did the three day cleanse using carrot juice and started on the mucous-less diet. All dairy and other animal products were removed from her diet and more raw food was added. After the cleanse she began taking the cleansing formulas **Lower Bowel** ,

Liver and Gallbladder and two months in she started on the **Blood Stream**. We rarely use the **Blood Stream** at the start of the program as we do not want to send too much to the liver until it has been strengthened by the formula **Liver and Gallbladder**.

We also stated her on the **Immucalm** formula which calmed her immune system down while still keeping it strong. This had the immediate result on diminishing the number of hives she was experiencing each day. She also used a salve we made from Comfrey, Plantain and Chickweed for soothing and healing the tender skin.

Because of the diet and the cleansing formulas with the **Immucalm**, the issue faded until all of her hives vanished. She has now moved forward with her learning and has just graduated from the Family Herbalist course at our clinic. She will make a wonderful herbalist in her home.

By the way, her family originally intervened to stop her from taking our treatments but now are so happy with the results they have put her back to work.

5.2   Betty – Multiple Sclerosis

As one of the most devastating illnesses we have dealt with at the clinic, we have also been overjoyed to see the amount of success using Dr. Christopher's protocols. Betty was a 33 year women who came into the clinic with advanced M.S. She was already dependent on a cane and her eyesight and voice were being affected. Her MRI showed three lesions on her brain and the prognosis was a long term progression towards a wheel chair.

As with all of these types of illnesses we prefer to follow Dr. Christopher's Incurables protocols. We presented her with the plan and she threw herself into the program. After the three day cleanse with carrot juice she immediately went vegan and quickly changed her diet over to about 80% raw, using mainly fresh fruits and vegetables. She also started the cleansing formulas of **Lower Bowel**, **Liver and Gallbladder** and the **Blood Stream** formula after two months.

To directly combat the M.S. she also starting taking the formulas **Immucalm** , **Relax-Eze** and the **Ear and Nerve**. As we stated before, due to this being an autoimmune issue, **Immucalm** calmed her immune system while allowing it to remain strong. While **Immucalm** does not cure M.S. every program should contain two prongs, one as a curative and the other as a palliative. The palliative is simply meant to make the patient comfortable while waiting for the cure to take effect. **Immucalm** allows the body to slow or stop the damage to the nervous system while the other formulas and diet are allowed to heal.

The formula **Relax-Eze** aids the body in calming and feeding the nervous system. The **Ear and Nerve** formula has been shown to be an excellent aid in healing the nerves and assisting with balance. She would use the **Ear and Nerve** each night in her ears before bed as well as taking it internally.

After just three weeks on the program she was able to put her cane away. As the months progressed, her balance improved to the point where she could wear high heals and was able to move out of her parents house for the first time in her life. She now holds down a job and is doing very well.

An UPDATE:

Recently, I have been performing reflexology treatments on Betty and with just three treatments to date she is already showing further improvement. Circulation is improving and what little numbness remained in her feet is completely disappearing.

An interesting side note is that we are finding in more and more cases that this issue as well as many others such as Lupus, RA, ALS, Parkensen's and many others are actually Lyme disease misdiagnosed. Please make sure to ask your doctor for further testing before you accept one of the above type of verdicts.

For those interested, we have a book published with Amazon titled *A Holistic Approach to Healing Lyme Disease.*

5.3   Matthew – Sigmoid Cancer

Matthew had been suffering with a Sigmoid tumor since 2009 and had already undergone one surgery for it as well as radiation. The radiation had destroyed his bladder and he was now using an external bag for the urine. Sadly, the cancer returned. Each year he had to receive a cat-scan and an MRI to watch the progression of the disease.

In 2013 he came into the clinic looking for an alternative solution to the medical industries drugs and radiation. He was somewhat reluctant to change his diet but we made it very clear that without a diet change, an issue of this manner would not be cured. He agreed and we began the program.

As with all cases such as this, he started with the three day cleanse using carrot juice. Carrot juice is one of the main juices to be used during any cancer program. Mixed with beet juice it is an excellent liver cleanser. We also started him immediately on the **Lower Bowel** as the cancer was in that area. 100% of the time cancer always starts in the bowels and is aggravated by a poorly functioning liver. The **Liver and Gallbladder** formula was also added.

While we normally only keep patients on the **Lower Bowel** and **Liver and Gallbladder** for three months total and the **Blood Stream** for one month at the end of the cleansing, in Matthew's case we kept him on the **Lower Bowel** and the **Blood Stream** formulas for most of the program. The reason for this is that cancer is always a condition of the bowels and therefore we wanted to keep the cleansing and healing properties of the **Lower Bowel** working the entire time. The **Blood Stream** was to aid in cleansing the blood of the cancer. While it was a cancer of the colon, the blood stream is always involved.

All of our cancer programs range from nine months to a year. This is to insure that the cancer has been eradicated. By the tenth month it came time for Matthew's yearly cat-scan and MRI. The good news came that there was no sign of the cancer spreading as seen from the cat-scan.

The MRI was inclusive to whether it could see any cancer. A final urine test was performed one year after we started the program and it came back negative. The colon cancer was gone.

Matthew of course was overjoyed as was I. It is very moving to see a patient recover from cancer without any more of the body being destroyed due to chemo and radiation therapies. He stated that he felt "normal" again for the first time in years.

5.4   Stacy – Polycystic Ovarian Syndrome

Polycystic Ovarian Syndrome affects approximately one out of fifteen women in the U.S. each year. As described in Wiki:

Polycystic ovary syndrome (PCOS), also called **hyperandrogenic anovulation (HA)**, or **Stein–Leventhal syndrome**, is a set of symptoms due to a hormone imbalance in women. Symptoms include: irregular or no menstrual periods, heavy periods, excess body and facial hair, acne, pelvic pain, trouble getting pregnant, and patches of thick, darker, velvety skin. Associated conditions include: type 2 diabetes, obesity, obstructive sleep apnea, heart disease, mood disorders, and endometrial cancer.

PCOS is due to a combination of genetic and environmental factors. Risk factors include obesity, not enough physical exercise, and a family history of someone with the condition. Diagnosis is based on two of the following three findings: no ovulation, high androgen levels, and ovarian cysts. Cysts may be detectable by ultrasound. Other conditions that produce similar symptoms include adrenal hyperplasia, hypothyroidism, and hyperprolactinemia.

PCOS has no cure. Treatment may involve lifestyle changes such as weight loss and exercise. Birth control pills may help with improving the regularity of periods, excess hair, and acne. Metformin and anti-androgens may also help. Other typical acne treatments and hair removal techniques may be used. Efforts to improve fertility include weight loss, clomiphene, or metformin. In vitro fertilization is used by some in whom other measures are not effective.

You will notice that it states there is no cure. The standard treatment plan is purely allopathic and uses birth control pills, which puts the woman at an increased risk of breast cancer. We are happy to report that Dr. Christopher was correct when he stated there is no incurable disease, only incurable people. Our case history here is about a patient of ours by the name of Stacy, who had, past tense, Polycystic Ovarian Syndrome, PCOS for short.

She came to our clinic at the age of 25 with a serious hormonal imbalance and excess hair growth.. She was also overweight and could not lose the extra pounds.

We ran the standard saliva and blood tests and it showed she had PCOS. Her previous physician had told her there was nothing she could do but take birth control pills to alleviate the symptoms, which did not work.

We put her on the standard program of **Lower Bowel**, and **Liver and Gallbladder** with the **Blood Stream** formula introduced later. She also started with a three day cleanse using carrot juice. She did notice a significant cleanse reaction of headaches and nausea while undergoing the cleanse.

To aid in the hormonal imbalance we started her on the formulas **Female Reproductive**, **Hormonal Changese**, wheatgerm oil and at least a quart of Red Raspberry tea each day, six days a week, one day off.

One of her other main complaints was Interstitial Cystitis, an inflammation of the lining of the bladder. For this she took the **Kidney** and **Bladder** formulas along with the **Soothing Digestion** combination. Within a week she began to notice the pain in her bladder was lessening. Overtime, this completely vanished.

We had to wait for her next cycle to occur but the good news came that it was somewhat better, with less pain and flow. Over the next three months her period completely normalized for the first time in her life.

One special note is that during this process she strictly followed the mucous-less diet and has to this day remained mostly raw. We have since run the same labs as before and her blood and saliva work shows no sign of the PCOS. An added benefit is that with all PCOS cases there is a serious issue with insulin resistance, hence making it difficult to lose the weight. For her, the insulin resistance completely disappeared and she has loss around forty pounds.

There is no such thing as an incurable disease...

5.5   James – Psoriasis/Genetic Issues

We have always considered James as one of our most special and well loved patients. He came to the clinic with one of the worst cases of psoriasis I have ever seen and was also afflicted with functional autism at the age of 35.

Below is an example of the stomach and back before we started treatment:

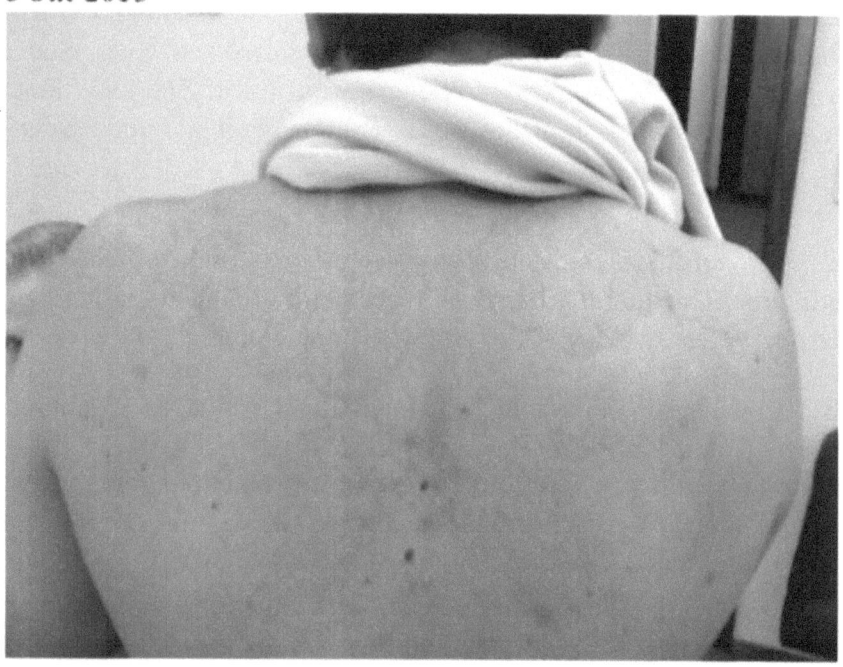

3 Jul 2013

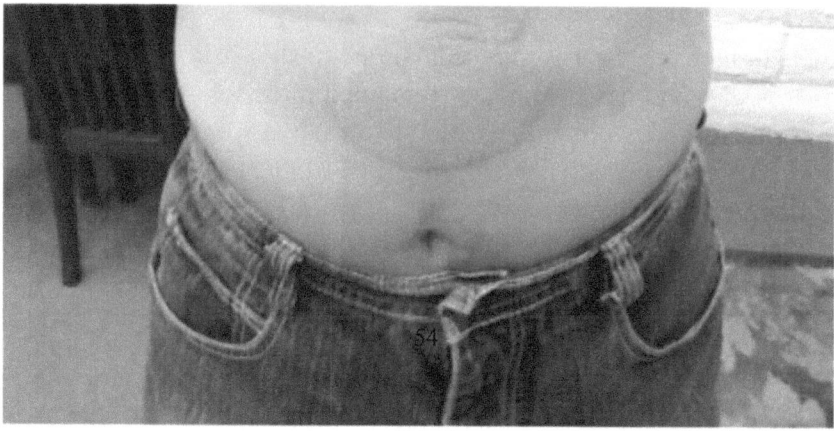

At first we mainly focused on the psoriasis and this is what his father had requested. Because this condition is an auto-immune disorder, we requested that James strictly follow the mucous-less diet. He did so wonderfully. Of all the patients who have crossed ours doors, he was the most accepting of the diet and never once complained. One of the things we do at the clinic is to supply our patients with a variety of sample menu plans and will even bring food into the clinic for them to try. This has been a great success as most folks are very nervous about changing their diets and have no idea where to start. By instructing them and taking time to teach, it can remove a significant amount of stress from the program.

We also recommended using the formulas **Lower Bowel, Liver and Gallbladder** and **Blood Stream.** You may notice that no matter what the condition or issue may be, there is a common vein found in all of them. This is the use of the cleansing formulas just listed above. Hippocrates stated to cleanse and nourish and Dr. Christopher taught us this as well. It has proven true time and again that if the body is cleansed it will uptake nutrients and natural medicines much faster. It is safe to say that 95% of all patients go through the three day cleanse and follow up using these formulas.

To work directly with the psoriasis we added the formulas **Complete Tissue and Bone** and **Immucalm**. Again, **Immucalm** calms the immune system while keeping it strong which helped slow the progress of the disease while the rest of the program worked on healing it.

Very quickly we began to notice a diminishing of the scales on his body. The itching vanished as well. But after about four months the progress came to a halt. The scales remained at a certain level and nothing I did seemed to aid the situation.

One day while James and his father were in the clinic we spoke about his disposition. His work place had complained about James's attitude and aggressive behaviors and had threatened to remove him from the county program. I knew that stress and emotions can have a serious affect on psoriasis so we ran a urinalysis for neurotransmitters. We had seen in the past that children with autism had a serious imbalance within the chemicals of the brain. The test came back very conclusive with indications of a propensity towards aggression and OCD (Obsessive Compulsive Disorder).

At this point we immediately went to work on the brain. We recommended the formulas **St. John's Wort**, **Relax-Eze** and **MindTrac**. We have seen amazing results with **St. John's Wort** as most patients in this condition have a serotonin imbalance. **St. John's Wort** works beautifully.

Relax-Eze calmed the nerves while feeding the brain. **MindTrac** worked specifically on the neurotransmitters. After just one month on this new regimen we ran another urinalysis for the neurotransmitters. The results were astounding. Every single neurotransmitter began to move towards the healthy range.

It was also at this time that we saw the greatest improvement in his psoriasis. Within a couple of months many of the spots completely disappeared with the rest showing a wonderful improvement.

Below is a recent picture of one of the worse spots he had originally displayed:

18 Mar 2015

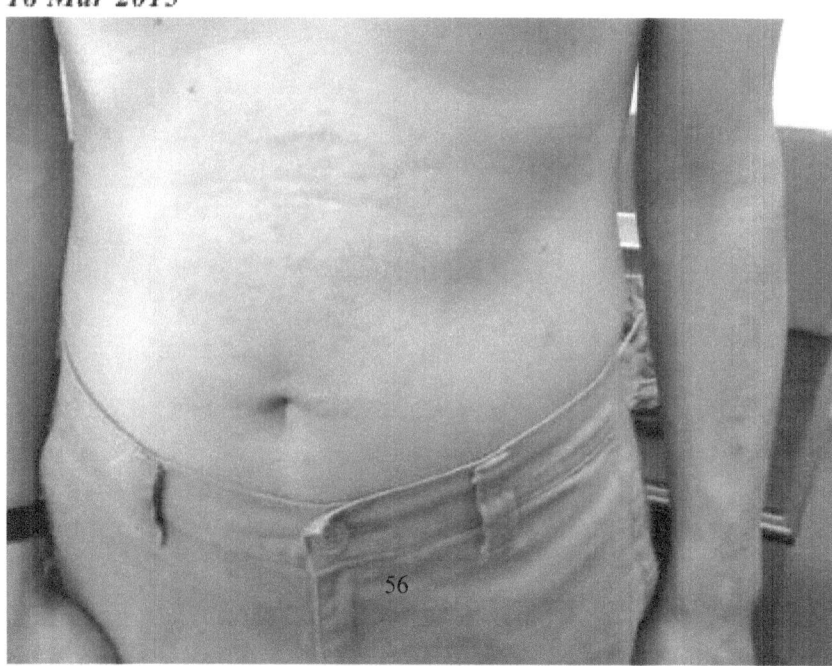

56

5.6 Robert – Type 1 Diabetes

Robert was a 35 year old patient with type 1 diabetes. This is the type considered incurable due to it's auto-immune character. He was morbidly obese weighing 362 pounds when he started the program. He also exhibited extensive foot neuropathy with severe skin abrasions due to the lack of healing. The nerves had died within the feet which made them feel like he was walking on blocks of wood. All his past healthcare providers had given up on him and claimed there was no hope. The disease would progress to the point where he would begin to lose his feet.

As with all patients we informed him there is no such thing as an incurable disease. He needed to take responsibility for his illness and to be a part of the cure. All any healthcare provider can do is to guide or teach the patient and to support them during the treatments. The cure is between the patient and what they believe in as a higher power.

As with all patients of this type of condition, he did the three cleanse with carrot juice and switched to the mucous-less diet. **Lower Bowel, Liver and Gallbladder , Blood Stream** and the **Kidney** formulas were incorporated into his daily regimen for six days a week with a day off and then repeat for months. We also added the **Pancreas** and **Immucalm** formulas to directly work with the condition.

All patients who follow the incurables program are informed this could take from nine months to a year to compete but that they should see some results within the first month. This was a wonderful example of that truth. Within the first three weeks on the program his amount of insulin used each day was cut in half and his blood sugar began to stabilize.

He was also able to report to his other primary a new and unexpected change. Never in his life had he seen any progress in slowing the disease. When he returned to his previous primary after six weeks she was shocked to find that the wounds were healing and that he was beginning to have feeling return to his feet. She quickly encouraged him to continue. He had lost approximately thirty pounds in that same period.

This type of progress continued until he was ready to take control of the disease and to manage it himself.

5.7   Nancy – Myasthenia Gravis

According to Wiki:

Myasthenia gravis (from Greek μῦς "muscle", ἀσθένεια "weakness", and Latin: *gravis* "serious"; abbreviated **MG**) is either an autoimmune or congenital neuromuscular disease that leads to fluctuating muscle weakness and fatigue. In the most common cases, muscle weakness is caused by circulating antibodies that block acetylcholine receptors at the postsynaptic neuromuscular junction, inhibiting the excitatory effects of the neurotransmitter acetylcholine on nicotinic receptors at neuromuscular junctions. Alternatively, in a much rarer form, muscle weakness is caused by a genetic defect in some portion of the neuromuscular junction, that is inherited at birth as opposed to developing it through autoimmunity later in life or through passive transmission by the mother's immune system at birth.

Myasthenia is treated medically with acetylcholinesterase inhibitors or immunosuppressants, and, in selected cases, thymectomy. The disease is diagnosed in 3 to 30 people per million per year. Diagnosis is becoming more common due to increased awareness. MG must be distinguished from congenital myasthenic syndromes that can present similar symptoms but do not respond to immunosuppressive treatments.

As you may notice, here again, this is considered incurable and is treated usually through immunosuppressants. These types of drugs leave the patient open to every bacteria, virus or fungus they may come into contact. The conventional medical community also perform a very serious surgery called thymectomy, where they remove the Thymus gland, one of the most important immune glands.

They perform these surgeries and prescribe these drugs because of the way they look at the auto-immune disease. They believe the body's immune system has lost control and begins to attack the body.

We do not believe this philosophy. We believe the immune system is working perfectly. In every type of auto-immune condition a particular cell type in the body is in a weaken state and does not display it's marker or flag which informs the immune system that it is part of self. The immune system therefore destroys the cell. Our protocol is to support the immune system while calming it down aiding the body in regrowing cells with the proper markers.

Our patient in this case was Nancy, a 34 year old woman with MG. She came to my attention right after graduating from the School of Natural Healing. I had turned in my financial paperwork to my CPA and Nancy was her secretary. When Nancy saw my paperwork and realized I was a natural, holistic healthcare provider she gave me a call. I informed her that I had just graduated but I would not turn her away. At that point we had not opened our first clinic. She was still willing, due to desperation, to see me. To protect ourselves legally, we opened our very first clinic to give us some type of umbrella with which to treat her. So I now had my first patient and she was of the most dangerous types of this condition.

During her first visit she asked for an exam to show us the scar from the thymectomy. She was also on Imuran and Prednisone and was told she would be on these for the rest of her life. She was also informed that the thymectomy failed and that she could have an MG crisis at any time. An MG crisis is when the patient attempts to breath but the signal is not received at the diaphragm.

As with any patient with the classic incurable tag, I inform them that they will be looking at a nine month to a year program. She would also be required to go on the mucous -less diet with a progression towards a significant portion of it being raw. The three day cleanse was also recommended.

With good faith she completed the cleanse and began the diet. She started on the basic formulas **Lower Bowel** , **Liver and Gallbladder**, **Blood Stream** and **Kidney**. We also added the formulas **Immuncalm** , **Complete Tissue and Bone** and **Ear and Nerve**. The **Complete Tissue and Bone** was added to aid in rebuilding the muscle and nerve tissues while the **Ear and Nerve** was very specific to the nerve regrowth. **Relax-Eze** was also added for nerve regrowth and to calm them.

She never did have an MG crisis during the program, which for her only lasted nine months. Due to her age she was able to heal more quickly than some of the older patients. In that short period of time she was able to get off of the Imuran and Prednisone.

Sixteen years ago I could not do the lab work I can today so I recommended she return to her previous primary and get a series of labs done to see what her present condition might show. When the labs were completed her physician looked at her with a stunned looked on his face and remarked that she must be in remission. To him she could not possibly be cured. At this point I told her she was through with the program and to simply watch her diet and follow healthy lifestyle choices.

We kept the clinic open for some time before we moved toward the west coast. Seven years past when I received a letter from the IRS claiming a $200 error on my taxes from back in the days when I was using my old CPA. I got on the phone and called her and to my great joy Nancy answered the phone.

We are very informal at our clinic and we are all on a first name basis. I happily exclaimed Nancy and she responded with yelling Earendil. I asked how she was doing after seven years and she proudly informed me that the disease never did return.

This is the reason I do what I do.

5.8 Cathy – Epstein Barr

One of the most common disorders in this society is chronic fatigue syndrome. It is usually caused by either a serious Candida overgrowth or by an Epstein Barr viral infection. It is also considered incurable. Most physicians will not even test for it because they feel it is a waste of time to check for something they cannot "fix".

Cathy was a 55 year old woman with confirmed Epstein Barr. This brought on extensive fatigue to the point she had difficulty getting out of bed before 10:00 or 11:00 in the morning. This caused a significant amount of stress as she ran her own business and this impacted her ability to perform the basic tasks the work required. It also caused muscle and joint pain similar to arthritis.

She completed the three day cleanse using apple juice and switched to a vegan diet. We also started her on **Lower Bowel, Liver and Gallbladder** and later, **Blood Stream**. To directly combat the virus we recommended significant doses of Garlic along with Echinacea and Goldenseal. **Immucalm** was added to calm her immune system. The **Joint** formula was also used as an aid for the joint and muscle pains.

Within the first month she began to notice she had a little bit more energy and was not sleeping as late. Her joint pain also began to diminish. Within a total of six months all of the fatigue had vanished and she was awakening refreshed by 5:00 or 6:00 in the morning. We ran a final Epstein Barr blood test and it came back negative.

I still see her running her company for the various grocery stores in our area and she always has a smile on her face.

5.9   Carol – Hysterectomy at age 27

Currently in the United States there are approximately 200,000 hysterectomies a year and I would be willing to say that is about 200,000 too many. One of the most memorable cases was a young lady who came to us at the age of 27.

She had been suffering from endometriosis and her other doctor had already had one ovary removed and was pushing for the other, along with her uterus and cervix. Her parents knew me and tried to get her to come into the clinic before the final surgery. Alas, they did not convince her and she went ahead and had everything else removed.

She eventually did come to the clinic as a patient but this was three months post-OP and 5 foot five inches and 85 pounds, pale as a sheet and addicted to Vicodin the pain killer prescribed for after surgery care. She was in tears as she felt no one would care to marry her since she could not have children and the previous doctor had told her she would have to wear an Estrogen patch the rest of her life. Needless to say there was little I could do to help with the baby issue but I told her she would be able to avoid the hormone replacement therapy. She was skeptical as she believed all estrogen came form the ovaries but I explained to her that the liver was also capable of producing it if in a healthy state. She decided to give our program a try.

We ran a hormone panel before treatment which was able to give us a "before" snapshot of her state. She then changed her diet to a healthy vegan based one and did a candida cleanse to prepare her immune system. This also allowed her to better assimilate her foods and then medications we gave her. After it was completed we stated her on the same program as mentioned earlier with patients with PCOS using herbs such as Red Raspberry tea, Blessed Thistle, Ginseng, Licorice root, False Unicorn, Sarsaparilla and Black Cohosh. She also continued to do colon and liver cleanses as well.

Within three months she was back up to 110 pounds, brown skin and no longer on Vicodin. We ran a three month hormone panel and without any hormone replacement therapy her Estrogen, Progesterone and Testosterone were back up within the normal ranges. She no longer had to take any of our medications.

Follow ups showed she never did experience any of the normal menopausal symptoms for women who have had a complete hysterectomy. She was instructed to stay on a healthy, vegan diet and to continue to take her Red Raspberry Tea on a daily basis.

5.10   Samuel – Chronic system wide body rash

It is sad to me when a patient comes into the clinic after months or years of suffering due to the fact they were never properly diagnosed. Following is one such case.

Samuel was a 58 year old male who presented with a rash from his head to his feet and had been suffering from it for the past nine months. The previous three months before we had our first appointment he had spent sitting in a chair or in bed as any movement caused it to flare up into an intense, maddening itch. He had gone to doctor after doctor including specialists such as dermatologist and even had skin punch biopsies done, to no avail for a diagnosis. His quality of life was at an all-time low and he had lost hope for a cure.

I went over his intake form and did what any good doctor would do and that is to try and find the root cause, not just treat the symptoms. I inquired as to what may have happened or changed in his life about nine or ten months ago. The only thing he could think of is that he had his mercury fillings removed just before the rash appeared. He described the procedure the dentist used. I discussed with the patient that the wrong procedure was done and that the mercury vapor had been inhaled and swallowed during the dental office visit.

Ingesting or inhaling mercury is like taking a massive dose of an antibiotic. It will destroy your bacterial micro-flora and leave you open to a massive candida overgrowth. I told him the rash was Candida Vasculitis, very common after such an event.

As with all of our chronic patients, the first thing we do is the 18 day candida cleanse. As mentioned earlier, this utilize a healthy, non-inflammatory vegan diet with herbal medications such as Black Walnut and Pau'd Arco for eliminating the yeast. We also employ the use of Slippery Elm bark and Licorice root for soothing and healing the intestinal walls, so inflamed from the yeast overgrowth.

By the end of the 18 days, his body wide rash had shrunk to a small patch on his upper left arm. He stated he was feeling wonderful and his energy was much improved. I started him on a heavy metal detox using Dr. Christopher's Bugle Heavy Metal formula and he remained on the diet to allow his body a chance to heal while the chelation continued.

After a total of two months he no longer experienced any sign of the rashes and the detox was completed. He and his wife continued to be patients with the clinic for various other minor issues for a couple of years and the rash never made another appearance.

5.11   Kim – Inoperable colon/appendix cancer

The cancer rate statistics in the year 1900 was 1 out 50 would have this disease sometime in their lifetime. By the 1970's, the start of the "war on Cancer", the rate was up to 1 out of 10. Today it has grown to 1 out 2 people in the United States will experience cancer sometime in their lifetime. Needless to say, the war on cancer is not being won.

At our clinic we have seen many. Many cases of cancer and the number of patients presenting this illness is on the rise within our practice. One particular case stands out as one of my patients to have had the joy and privilege to know.

She was a 59 year old woman who originally came to the clinic to be treated for psoriasis. During her initial appointment she asked if I would check on lump on her lower right abdomen. I told her I would be happy to check. She stated her other doctor had checked and dismissed it as a simply fatty deposit but her heart told her different. When we were going over her treatment plan for the psoriasis I lead her and her husband into the exam room.

I have been around quite a bit of cancer in my 20+ years of practice and as soon as I palpated the area I knew what it was. But, I kept the traditional poker face and suggested we check with ultrasound. We have ultrasound at the clinic so it was a simple matter of setting the machine up and within five minutes we were scanning the site. Her entire abdominal cavity was full of what appeared to be tumors and acites (fluid filled pockets often caused by cancer in the bowels and appendix).

The poker face was gone and she could see there was some concern. I requested we get some blood work done to get a better idea. She agreed and when the lab results came in it confirmed a 95% likelihood of cancer. She became very upset with her doctor dismissing her since at this point she had lost two months of possible treatment time. She returned to them and showed them our results. At this point the other doctor panicked and reran all of my tests and found the same results. The final diagnosis was colon and appendix cancer with Pseudomyxoma peritonei (PMP) .She was staged at stage four.

Or course, the recommended treatment plan from them was to surgically bulk the cancer and to run a very risky chemo therapy treatment that requires extensive blood transfusions. As a Jehovah Witness she was not able to accept the treatment. The other doctors told her she would be dead in six months if she did not take the chemotherapy. She still refused and returned to our clinic for a holistic program.

As with all chronic patients, the first step was the candida cleanse. Again, this is done to aid in healing the immune system. Cancer is a systemic failure of the immune system and it is a well established fact that it is important for the patient's own immune system to begin to fight back. Normally, most people are exposed to cancer as tiny little errant cells. In a healthy immune system we respond to the threat and destroy the cancer cells on our own. In the case of cancer patients, their immune system was compromised and did not destroy the threat.

This can have a wide variety of root causes but in the end we ALWAYS and with no exceptions, find each cancer patient presenting extensive candida overgrowth. It is our job then, at the beginning, to aid the patient in reestablishing the intestinal environment. Once this is done than the patient has a higher likelihood of having a stronger immune system.

Once the 18 day candida cleanse is completed we then proceed with actually fighting the cancer. The patient remains on a vegan diet but at this point they begin to increase dramatically the percentage of raw, live food. We supply them with a wide variety of meal plans, recipes and nutrition charts so this does not become a boring diet.

We also being the holistic medication portion of the regimen. Colon and liver cleanses are done throughout the program along with herbal formulas utilizing Poke root, Red Raspberry tea, Milk thistle, blood cleanser formulas using Red Clover, and Thunder god vine root.

Thunder god vine root has been studied extensively out of China, Germany and even here in the states under Johns Hopkins University. Clinical trial studies seem to indicate that this herb out of China is able to begin the process of apoptosis with in 40 days. Apoptosis is the process by which cancer cells switch off their DNA and "commit suicide", so to speak.

With programs such as this kind, we ask the patient to return to the clinic once a month so we can check their progress, run vitals, run tests in house, all in an effort to monitor their treatments. We also regularly ran blood work on her cancer markers.

With each visit she reported feeling better and the masses, examined through ultrasound continued to shrink. Her cancer marker also continued to drop closer to the normal ranges. MRIs and CT scans were run about every six months.

At her last MRI scan along with ultrasound and blood work the local hospital declared no sign of the cancer any longer and to their surprise, her colon had "rebuilt itself".

Something we try and teach each patient is that he body is an amazing creation and that it is designed with a built in "blueprint" if given the opportunity, it will heal and repair itself. As a very famous Naturopathic doctor and Master herbalist, Dr. John Christopher, stated:

"There is not such thing as an incurable disease, only incurable people".

About The Author

Dr. Earendil M. Spindelilus D.N.M., M.H., C.R. - Traditional Naturopath, Holistic Practitioner, Clinical Master Herbalist, Certified Nutritionist, Certified Reflexology, Member of Plant Savers of America, Member of American Botanical Council.

I hold a Doctorate degree in Natural Medicine. I have also been a lecturer since 1999. Board Certified Diplomate of Natural Medicine. Member of the American Council of Holistic Medicine.

I have always had a deep and abiding interest in the Plant Kingdom. Even very young I loved the way the herbs held the mystery of healing within them and how I could learn about them. I traveled around the world learning from different cultures their own unique floras and how they incorporated them into their daily lives. With each new herb I learned how special the world is and how Nature supplies us with all we need. In the 1990s I decided to take my education further and enrolled in the School and Natural Healing, the College of Herbal Medicine. I graduated in 1999 with my Master Herbalist. I have also studied with the New Eden School of Natural Medicine where I completed my Doctorate in Natural Medicine. To date, my wife and I have run two medical centers for natural healing. It has always been a great joy meeting with our patients. We are all meant to live a happy, healthy life and when we allow our body to perform it's innate ability to heal itself then this can happen. I am also a past board member of the Reflexology Association of California as well as a published author/writer of numerous holistic books and articles. I am also a past host of a holistic radio show. We currently run a Holistic YouTube channel.

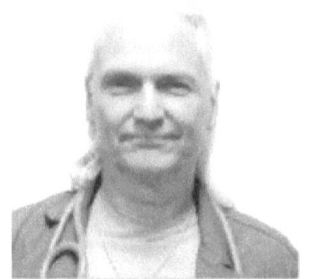